Life Reimagined: Thriving After A Serious Medical Condition

Antonio Savaro Champion

The Antonio Champion Story

Copyright © **Antonio Savaro**

All rights reserved. No part of this publication may be reproduced, distributed, or transmitted in any form or by any means, including photocopying, recording, or other electronic or mechanical methods, without the prior written permission of the publisher, except in the case of brief quotations embodied in critical reviews and certain other noncommercial uses permitted by copyright law.

Table of Contents

Chapter 1: The Early Years 5

Chapter 2: Growing Pains and Dreams in Brooklyn 11

Chapter 3: A Move to Atlanta: New Beginnings 21

Chapter 4 The First Diagnosis: Diabetes 28

Chapter 5: Life's Curveball: Heart Attack 33

Chapter 6: Pancreatitis: Another Challenge 42

Chapter 7: The Power of Family 51

Chapter 8: Brotherly Love 60

Chapter 9: Strength and Resilience 67

Chapter 10: A New Beginning for Antonio 70

Antonio's Daily Routine for Health Management 77

Conclusion: Reflection and Future Outlook 84

Antonio's Commitment to Long-Term Health..........91

Inspirational Message for Others..............................94

A Brighter Future...97

Conclusion...98

Chapter 1: The Early Years

Born in Gainesville, Georgia, in 1976, my early years were filled with the innocence of childhood and the dreams that only a young boy could imagine. Growing up in a small southern town, life was simple, but it wasn't without its challenges. My parents were hard-working people, striving to give my siblings and me the best life possible. Sadly, their journey ended too soon, leaving us to fend for ourselves much earlier than expected.

In Gainesville, family and community were everything. I remember the warm summer nights filled with the sounds of crickets and the laughter of neighbors. Those were the days when the world felt both incredibly large and intimately small, where everyone knew everyone, and the sense of community was as thick as the southern humidity.

As a young boy, my days were spent exploring the vast open fields and dense woods that surrounded our home. I would climb trees, chase fireflies, and build forts. Each day was a new adventure, filled with the wonders of nature and the boundless imagination of childhood.

School was a place of learning and socializing, but it was also where I first encountered the harsh realities of life. Bullying was a constant challenge, and I quickly learned the importance of standing up for myself and others. Despite the difficulties, I found solace in my studies and the friendships I formed along the way.

My mom instilled in me the values of integrity and perseverance. I lost my mother at the age of 15, due to complications of being a noncompliant diabetic and heart problems.

The loss of my parents was a turning point in my life. It was a tragedy that forced my siblings and me to grow up quickly and take on responsibilities far beyond our years. Stacy, my youngest sister, became the anchor of our family, along with my other sisters Renea and Kathy, while my brothers Bilal and Meco were still teens at the time of our mother loss. Together, we navigated the challenges of life without the guidance of our parents.

The summers in Gainesville were hot and humid, but they were also a time of freedom and exploration. I would spend hours over at my cousins house playing and riding bikes. It was a place of tranquility, where I could escape the worries of the world and simply be a kid.

As I grew older, I began to take on odd jobs knowing I wanted better for myself. Whether it was mowing lawns, delivering newspapers, or working at the local grocery store, I learned the value of hard work and the satisfaction that came from earning my own money. These experiences taught me important life skills and shaped my work ethic.

Despite the challenges, there were moments of joy and celebration. Family gatherings were filled with laughter, music, and delicious food. My sister Stacy fried chicken was legendary, and her home was always filled with the comforting aroma of southern cooking. These gatherings were a reminder of the importance of family and the bonds that held us together.

Education was a priority for me, and I was determined to make the most of the opportunities I had. I excelled in my studies and took pride in my achievements. My teachers recognized my potential and encouraged me to pursue my dreams, instilling in me a belief that I could achieve anything I set my mind to.

The sense of community in Gainesville was a constant source of support. Neighbors looked out for one another, and there was always someone willing to lend a helping hand. This sense of belonging gave me the confidence to face the challenges that came my way and the assurance that I was never truly alone.

Music played a significant role in my life, providing a soundtrack to my experiences. From the soulful tunes of Motown to the rhythmic beats of hip-hop, music was a source of inspiration and solace. I would spend hours listening to records and dreaming of a future filled with possibilities.

As I approached my teenage years, the world began to change. The small-town life I had known started to give way to new opportunities and challenges. The innocence of childhood began to fade, and I found myself grappling with the complexities of adolescence.

Through it all, my family remained my anchor. Stacy continued to be a guiding force, while Bilal and Meco provided unwavering support. My nieces and nephews brought joy and laughter into our lives, reminding us of the importance of staying connected and cherishing the moments we had together.

The lessons I learned during those early years in Gainesville have stayed with me throughout my life. They taught me the importance of resilience, the value of hard work, and the power of family and community. These experiences shaped the person I would become and laid the foundation for the j

Chapter 2: Growing Pains and Dreams in Brooklyn

Moving to Brooklyn, New York, was like stepping into a different universe. The bustling streets, the towering buildings, and the diverse cultures all seemed overwhelming at first. But soon, Brooklyn became home. It was here that my dreams began to take shape and my personality started to shine.

The challenges of growing up in a big city were real. The temptations and the pressures were ever-present. But amidst the chaos, I found solace in my family and my best friend Rico. Rico and I had been inseparable since childhood, and our bond only grew stronger as we navigated the maze of city life together.

Brooklyn was a melting pot of cultures, with people from all walks of life coming together in one vibrant borough. The diversity was both a source of fascination and a challenge. I quickly learned to appreciate the different backgrounds and perspectives that surrounded me, and this cultural exposure broadened my horizons in ways I couldn't have imagined.

Our neighborhood in Brooklyn was a bustling hive of activity. Street vendors peddled their goods, children played on the sidewalks, and the constant hum of traffic was a backdrop to daily life. It was a far cry from the quiet, small-town life I had known in Gainesville, but it was exhilarating in its own way.

Rico and I explored every corner of our new neighborhood. Whether it was finding the best pizza joint or discovering a hidden basketball court, we made Brooklyn our playground. Rico's energy and adventurous spirit were contagious, and together, we embraced the excitement of city life.

School in Brooklyn was a mix of excitement and intimidation. The sheer size of the student body was overwhelming at first, but I soon found my footing. I made friends who shared my interests and passions, and we bonded over our love of sports, music, and the dream of a better future. These friendships became a source of strength and inspiration.

One of the most significant adjustments was learning to navigate the subway system. The maze of tunnels and trains seemed daunting, but over time, I became a master of the New York City transit system. The subway became a symbol of my growing independence and my ability to adapt to new challenges.

Our apartment in Brooklyn was small but cozy. It was a place where our family gathered after long days, sharing meals and stories. Stacy took on the role of caretaker, ensuring that our home was always filled with love and warmth. Her strength and resilience were a guiding force for all of us.

The streets of Brooklyn became our playground. Rico and I spent countless hours playing basketball at the local park, honing our skills and dreaming of making it big. The camaraderie and competition on the court taught us valuable lessons about teamwork, discipline, and perseverance.

Despite the many distractions and temptations, I remained focused on my education. I knew that doing well in school was my ticket to a better future. My teachers recognized my potential and encouraged me to aim high. Their belief in me was a constant source of motivation.

Music was a constant presence in my life. The sounds of hip-hop and R&B echoed through the streets, and I found solace in the beats and lyrics that spoke to my experiences. Music became an outlet for my emotions and a way to connect with others who shared my love for the art form.

The sense of community in Brooklyn was different from what I had known in Gainesville, but it was just as strong. Neighbors looked out for one another, and there was a sense of solidarity among the residents. We were all in this together, navigating the challenges of city life and supporting each other along the way.

My siblings and I faced our share of struggles, but we always found a way to overcome them. Bilal and Meco were my partners in crime, and together, we navigated the complexities of adolescence. Whether it was dealing with bullies or finding ways to make extra money, we had each other's backs.

Stacy was our anchor, always ensuring that we stayed on the right path. Her guidance and support were unwavering, and she made countless sacrifices to provide for us. She was a role model and a source of inspiration, showing us the importance of hard work and dedication.

Brooklyn offered opportunities that I had never imagined. I joined after-school programs and community organizations that opened doors to new experiences. These programs allowed me to explore my interests, develop new skills, and build a network of mentors and supporters.

As I grew older, I began to take on part-time jobs to help support our family. Whether it was working at the corner store or delivering newspapers, I learned the value of hard work and the importance of responsibility. These experiences taught me important life skills and shaped my character.

The pressure to succeed was ever-present, but it was also a driving force. I was determined to make the most of the opportunities I had and to create a better future for myself and my family. This determination fueled my efforts in both academics and extracurricular activities.

The streets of Brooklyn were filled with both danger and opportunity. I witnessed the harsh realities of life in the city, but I also saw the resilience and determination of the people who called it home. These experiences shaped my worldview and taught me the importance of perseverance and hope.

Our family gatherings in Brooklyn were filled with laughter, music, and delicious food. These moments were a reminder of the importance of staying connected and cherishing the time we had together. My nieces and nephews brought joy and energy into our lives, reminding us of the beauty of family.

Brooklyn was a place of dreams and possibilities. The skyline of Manhattan served as a constant reminder of the potential for greatness. I often found myself gazing at the towering buildings, imagining the future that awaited me. These dreams fueled my ambition and motivated me to keep pushing forward.

The diversity of Brooklyn exposed me to different cultures, traditions, and ways of life. This exposure broadened my horizons and made me more open-minded and accepting of others. It was a valuable lesson in the importance of diversity and the strength that comes from embracing different perspectives.

My experiences in Brooklyn taught me the importance of resilience and adaptability. The challenges I faced helped me develop a strong sense of self and the ability to overcome obstacles. These qualities would prove invaluable in the years to come as I navigated the ups and downs of life.

The support of my family was a constant source of strength. No matter what challenges we faced, we knew we could rely on each other. Stacy, Bilal, and Meco were my rock, and their love and encouragement gave me the confidence to pursue my dreams.

As I approached the end of high school, the future was filled with both excitement and uncertainty. I knew that college was my next step, but I was also aware of the challenges that lay ahead. The experiences and lessons I had gained in Brooklyn had prepared me for this new chapter, and I was ready to take on the world.

Brooklyn was more than just a place; it was a transformative experience that shaped who I was and who I would become. The memories, friendships, and lessons from my time in the city were etched into my soul, and they would continue to guide me on my journey.

As I embarked on the next chapter of my life, I carried with me the strength, resilience, and determination that I had cultivated in Brooklyn. The dreams that had taken shape in the city were now ready to be realized, and I was prepared to face whatever challenges

Chapter 3: A Move to Atlanta: New Beginnings

The decision to move to Atlanta marked a significant turning point in my life. Leaving behind the familiarity of Brooklyn and embarking on a new journey in the South was both exciting and daunting. Atlanta, with its rich history and vibrant culture, offered a fresh start and new opportunities.

The drive from Brooklyn to Atlanta was long, filled with anticipation and reflections on the past. As I crossed state lines and approached Georgia, the excitement for what lay ahead began to overshadow any lingering doubts. I couldn't wait to see what the future held for us in this new city.

Atlanta greeted us with its sprawling skyline and the warmth of Southern hospitality. The city was a blend of modernity and tradition, with skyscrapers towering over historic neighborhoods. It was a place where the past and present coexisted harmoniously, and I was eager to become a part of it.

My new neighborhood in Atlanta was welcoming and diverse. The sense of community was palpable, and neighbors greeted us with open arms. The transition from the fast-paced life of Brooklyn to the more relaxed atmosphere of Atlanta took some getting used to, but it also provided a sense of peace and stability.

Settling into my new home was a family affair. Purchased with cash from my niece Courtney was instrumental in making the transition smooth. I spent days unpacking, arranging furniture, and adding personal touches to make the space feel like mine. The process was truly a lasting bond with me and my family.

Exploring Atlanta became an adventure in itself. From the bustling streets of downtown to the serene parks and historic landmarks, there was always something new to discover. I would often set out on spontaneous excursions, eager to uncover the hidden gems of our new city.

One of the highlights of my move was discovering the rich musical heritage of Atlanta. The city was a hub for hip-hop and R&B, and the local music scene was thriving. I immersed myself in the sounds and rhythms that defined the city's identity. Music events and local performances became my regular outings.

The change of pace in Atlanta also allowed for deeper connections with my family. We spent more quality time together, sharing meals, stories, and laughter. Stacy continued to be the guiding force, ensuring that our home was filled with love and support. Bilal and Courtney were my constant companions, always ready for a new adventure or a heart-to-heart conversation.

Atlanta's diverse culinary scene was a treat for the senses. From soul food to international cuisines, the city's food culture was a testament to its melting-pot identity. Family dinners became an opportunity to explore new flavors and bond over shared meals. My nieces and nephews loved trying new dishes, and their enthusiasm was contagious.

The move to Atlanta also marked a period of personal growth. The new environment encouraged me to step out of my comfort zone and embrace new challenges. I joined clubs and organizations, made new friends, and pursued interests that I hadn't explored before. The supportive community and the city's vibrant energy fueled my ambitions.

The sense of community in Atlanta was a source of strength. Neighbors looked out for one another, and there was a genuine spirit of unity. Whether it was a neighborhood barbecue, a community clean-up, or a local festival, there were always opportunities to connect and contribute.

As I settled into life in Atlanta, I found myself reflecting on the journey that had brought me here. The challenges and triumphs of Brooklyn had shaped me, but Atlanta was where I would forge my path forward. The city's dynamic culture, supportive community, and endless opportunities made it the perfect place to pursue my dreams.

Our family continued to grow stronger in Atlanta. Stacy's unwavering support and guidance, Courtney's constant companionship, and the joy brought by my nieces and nephews created a foundation of love and resilience. Together, we faced the challenges of our new environment and celebrated the milestones along the way.

The move to Atlanta also brought new opportunities for personal and academic growth. The supportive school environment, combined with the city's resources and networks, opened doors to new experiences. I took advantage of internships, volunteer opportunities, and extracurricular activities that enriched my education and personal development.

Atlanta's rich history and cultural significance were a source of inspiration. The city had been at the forefront of the civil rights movement, and its legacy of activism and social justice resonated deeply with me. I became involved in community initiatives and advocacy efforts, determined to contribute to positive change in my new home.

I was filled with a sense of accomplishment and anticipation. The move to Atlanta had been a transformative experience, shaping my identity and aspirations. The support of my family, the friendships I had built, and the lessons I had learned prepared me for the next chapter of my life.

Reflecting on the journey, I realized that the move to Atlanta had been more than just a change of location. It had been a journey of self-discovery, growth, and resilience. The challenges we faced had strengthened our bonds, and the opportunities we embraced had shaped our futures. Atlanta had become more than just a city; it was home.

Chapter 4 The First Diagnosis: Diabetes

Antonio was a man of routine, a lover of life's little pleasures. He balanced his demanding job with regular workouts and a nutritious diet, always making sure to take care of his health. His friends often joked that he was the picture of health and vitality. That was until the autumn of his 35th year, when his life took an unexpected turn.

It all started with small, seemingly insignificant changes. Antonio found himself making frequent trips to the bathroom and drinking more water than usual. He brushed it off as nothing more than stress and the remnants of a particularly busy summer. But as the weeks went on, the symptoms didn't abate; they intensified. He was losing weight despite his hearty appetite, and there was a persistent fatigue that no amount of sleep could shake off.

One crisp October morning, driven by a nagging concern, Antonio decided to visit his doctor. The check-up seemed routine until the doctor mentioned checking his blood sugar levels. The prick of the needle was small, but the result was monumental. Antonio had diabetes.

Antonio sat in stunned silence, the doctor's words echoing in his mind. Diabetes. How could it be? He had always taken such good care of himself. The reality of the diagnosis crashed over him like a wave, bringing with it a flood of emotions. Fear, disbelief, and a deep, gnawing worry about what this meant for his future.

The days following his diagnosis were a whirlwind of appointments and information.

Antonio felt like he was drowning in a sea of medical terms and lifestyle changes. There was so much to learn, so many adjustments to make. The thought of injecting insulin and constantly monitoring his blood sugar levels was daunting. The fear of potential complications loomed large, casting a shadow over his thoughts.

But Antonio was not alone in his journey. His family and friends rallied around him, their concern palpable but their support unwavering. They helped him navigate the maze of information, offering encouragement and a shoulder to lean on. His healthcare team provided him with a comprehensive plan, outlining the changes he needed to make in his diet, exercise routine, and daily habits.

The first few weeks were the hardest. Antonio struggled with the new routine, the constant pricks of the needle, and the meticulous tracking of his blood sugar levels. There were moments of frustration and self-doubt, but he pushed through, determined to take control of his health. His counselor played a crucial role, helping him manage the emotional toll of living with a chronic condition.

As time went on, Antonio adapted to his new reality. Monitoring his blood sugar levels became second nature, and he developed a balanced diet and exercise routine that worked for him. He found solace in a support group, connecting with others who shared similar experiences. Their stories and insights provided him with a sense of community and understanding that he had been craving.

Through it all, Antonio maintained a positive outlook. He celebrated the small victories – a well-managed blood sugar level, a new favorite healthy recipe, a particularly good day. He focused on the progress he had made and the improvements in his health, rather than the limitations imposed by his condition.

Antonio's journey with diabetes was not easy, but it was one of growth and resilience. It taught him the importance of self-care, the value of a strong support system, and the power of a positive mindset. His experience served as a reminder that, with determination and the right support, it is possible to manage a chronic condition and lead a fulfilling life. Antonio hoped that his story would inspire and encourage others facing similar challenges to take charge of their health and never lose hope.

Chapter 5: Life's Curveball: Heart Attack

Just when I thought I had a handle on my diabetes, life threw me another curveball. It was an ordinary day, filled with routine activities and the usual hustle and bustle. I had just finished a workout and was preparing dinner when I suddenly felt an intense pain in my chest. It was like nothing I had ever experienced before. My heart felt like it was being squeezed, and I struggled to catch my breath. Panic set in as I realized something was terribly wrong.

Stacy called 911, and within minutes, an ambulance arrived. The paramedics worked swiftly, hooking me up to monitors and administering medication. The ride to Piedmont Hospital was a blur of sirens and flashing lights. I remember feeling a sense of detachment, as if I were watching the scene unfold from outside my body. Fear gripped me, and I couldn't help but wonder if this was the end.

At Piedmont Hospital, doctors confirmed my worst fear: I had suffered a heart attack. The news was devastating. I was immediately taken to the cardiac unit for further tests and treatment. The next few days were a whirlwind of procedures and medical jargon. I underwent an angioplasty to open blocked arteries, and the doctors placed stents to keep the blood flowing. Additionally, I received a defibrillator implant to help regulate my heart rhythm. The experience was surreal, and I felt like I was living in a nightmare.

The recovery process was grueling. I spent a month at Piedmont Hospital, receiving round-the-clock care from the dedicated medical staff. I was weak and exhausted, both physically and emotionally. The reality of my condition began to sink in, and I struggled with feelings of vulnerability and helplessness. But through it all, my family was by my side. Stacy, Bilal, Meco, and the rest of my family took turns staying with me, offering their unwavering support and encouragement.

One of the hardest parts of the recovery was the lifestyle changes I had to make. The doctors emphasized the importance of a heart-healthy diet, regular exercise, and stress management. I had already made significant changes to manage my diabetes, but now I had to be even more diligent. It felt overwhelming, but I knew it was necessary for my health and well-being.

Stacy once again took the lead, researching heart-healthy recipes and helping me create a meal plan that worked for my lifestyle. We experimented with new ingredients and cooking methods, discovering that healthy eating didn't have to be bland or boring. Her dedication and love were a constant source of motivation.

Exercise became even more critical in my recovery. I started with gentle activities like walking and gradually increased the intensity as my strength returned. Bilal and Meco often joined me, turning our workouts into bonding sessions. Their support and encouragement made the process less daunting and more enjoyable.

Stress management was another crucial aspect of my recovery. I learned the importance of mindfulness and relaxation techniques. Meditation, deep breathing exercises, and yoga became part of my daily routine. These practices helped me manage stress and anxiety, improving my overall well-being.

Despite the challenges, there were moments of triumph and hope. Each day brought small victories, whether it was walking a little farther, cooking a new healthy recipe, or simply feeling a bit stronger. These achievements, no matter how small, fueled my determination to keep pushing forward.

The support of my family was unwavering. They were my rock, providing love, encouragement, and a sense of normalcy during a tumultuous time. Charity and Courtney, my nieces, often visited with handmade cards and drawings. Their innocence and positivity were a reminder of the beauty and resilience of life.

The heart attack also served as a wake-up call, forcing me to reevaluate my priorities and the way I lived my life. I realized the importance of taking care of my physical and mental health and the value of the relationships and connections that sustained me. This newfound perspective guided me as I navigated the road to recovery.

The experience also brought my family closer together. We became more open with each other, sharing our fears, hopes, and dreams. The bonds that held us together grew stronger, and we learned to lean on each other in times of need. This sense of unity was a source of strength and comfort.

As I progressed in my recovery, I began to reach out to others who had experienced similar health challenges. I joined support groups and shared my story, offering encouragement and hope to those who were just beginning their journey. Helping others became a way to give back and to find purpose in my own struggles.

The journey was not without its setbacks. There were days when I felt discouraged and overwhelmed by the demands of managing both diabetes and heart disease. But each setback taught me valuable lessons and made me more resilient. I learned to be patient with myself and to take each day as it came.

My faith remained a source of comfort and guidance. I found solace in prayer and meditation, and my connection to a higher power gave me the strength to face each day with hope and determination. My faith was a beacon of light in the darkest moments, providing a sense of peace and assurance.

The experience of having a heart attack was a stark reminder of the fragility of life. It made me appreciate the simple things and cherish every moment with my loved ones. I learned to savor every meal, enjoy every walk, and treasure the time spent with family and friends. This newfound appreciation for life was a gift that came from the adversity I had faced.

As I continued to recover, I set new goals for myself. I wanted to not only manage my health but to thrive and live a fulfilling life. I pursued interests and activities that brought me joy and fulfillment, whether it was playing music, volunteering in the community, or spending time with loved ones.

The experience also deepened my sense of empathy and compassion. I became more attuned to the struggles of others and more willing to offer support and encouragement. The journey had taught me the importance of kindness and connection, and I was determined to live by these values.

Reflecting on the journey, I realized that the heart attack had been a turning point in my life. It had forced me to confront my vulnerabilities and to make changes that improved my quality of life. It had brought my family closer together and had given me a new perspective on the importance of self-care and resilience.

The journey of recovering from a heart attack was a rollercoaster of emotions. There were moments of fear and uncertainty, but there were also moments of joy and triumph. Each day was a testament to my resilience and determination to live a healthy and fulfilling life.

As I looked to the future, I was filled with a sense of hope and determination. I knew that there would be challenges, but I also knew that I had the strength and support to overcome them. The experience of having a heart attack had made me stronger, and I was ready to continue thriving in life.

Chapter 6: Pancreatitis: Another Challenge

The pain was unlike anything I had ever experienced before. It started as a dull ache in my abdomen but quickly intensified into a sharp, relentless agony. I knew something was seriously wrong. Stacy rushed me to the emergency room, where doctors ran a series of tests. The diagnosis was pancreatitis. Hearing the news, my heart sank. I was immediately admitted to Emory University Hospital for further treatment.

The severity of my condition required intensive care, and I was placed in the ICU. The next few days were a blur of medical procedures, IV drips, and constant monitoring. The doctors were working tirelessly to stabilize my condition and manage the inflammation in my pancreas. The pain was relentless, but I found solace in knowing that I was in capable hands.

My stay at Emory University Hospital lasted four long months. It was a journey fraught with complications. During my time there, I battled a staph infection, E. coli, and pneumonia. Each setback felt like a blow to my spirit, but I refused to give up. The medical staff at Emory were dedicated and compassionate, providing the best care possible and offering words of encouragement when I needed them most.

The staph infection was particularly challenging. It required aggressive treatment with antibiotics and constant vigilance to prevent it from spreading. The infection left me feeling weak and vulnerable, but I knew I had to stay strong and keep fighting. The support of my family was a lifeline during this difficult time.

E. coli was another hurdle in my recovery. The infection caused severe gastrointestinal distress, adding to the already intense pain from pancreatitis. The doctors worked tirelessly to treat the infection and manage my symptoms. It was a grueling process, but I knew that each step brought me closer to recovery.

Pneumonia was the final blow in a series of health challenges. The infection made breathing difficult and left me feeling exhausted. The doctors provided oxygen therapy and medication to help clear my lungs and fight the infection. It was a slow and arduous process, but I remained determined to overcome this obstacle.

Throughout my stay at Emory, the support of my family was unwavering. Stacy, Bilal, and Meco took turns staying with me, providing comfort and encouragement. Their presence was a constant reminder that I was not alone in this fight. Charity and Courtney, my nieces, often visited with handmade cards, books, and different foods. Their innocence and positivity were a beacon of hope during the darkest moments.

Charity and Courtney's visits were a highlight of my days in the hospital. They would bring a variety of foods to tempt my appetite and books to keep my mind engaged. We would sit together, and they would read to me or share stories from their day. Their laughter and energy were infectious, and they provided a much-needed distraction from the pain and monotony of hospital life.

The experience of being in the ICU was both physically and emotionally draining. The constant beeping of monitors, the sterile hospital environment, and the uncertainty of my condition weighed heavily on me. But through it all, I remained focused on my recovery. I knew that I had to stay strong for myself and for my family.

One of the most significant challenges was maintaining a positive mindset. The pain and setbacks were overwhelming, but I made a conscious effort to focus on the progress I was making. Each small victory, whether it was a stable blood sugar level or a clear lung scan, was a step forward. These moments of progress fueled my determination to keep pushing forward.

The medical staff at Emory University Hospital were incredible. Their dedication, expertise, and compassion made a world of difference in my recovery. They provided not only medical care but also emotional support. Their words of encouragement and belief in my ability to overcome these challenges gave me the strength to keep fighting.

The road to recovery was long and arduous, but I learned valuable lessons along the way. I realized the importance of patience, resilience, and self-compassion. Each setback taught me to be kinder to myself and to appreciate the progress I was making, no matter how small.

Faith remained a source of comfort and guidance throughout my journey. I found solace in prayer and meditation, and my connection to a higher power gave me the strength to face each day with hope and determination. My faith was a beacon of light in the darkest moments, providing a sense of peace and assurance.

The experience also deepened my relationships with my family. We became more open and honest with each other, sharing our fears, hopes, and dreams. The bonds that held us together grew stronger, and we learned to lean on each other in times of need. This sense of unity was a source of strength and comfort.

As I began to recover, I set new goals for myself. I wanted to not only manage my health but to thrive and live a fulfilling life. I pursued interests and activities that brought me joy and fulfillment, whether it was playing music, volunteering in the community, or spending time with loved ones.

The experience also deepened my sense of empathy and compassion. I became more attuned to the struggles of others and more willing to offer support and encouragement. The journey had taught me the importance of kindness and connection, and I was determined to live by these values.

The journey of recovering from pancreatitis and the associated infections was a rollercoaster of emotions. There were moments of fear and uncertainty, but there were also moments of joy and triumph. Each day was a testament to my resilience and determination to live a healthy and fulfilling life.

Reflecting on the journey, I realized that the challenges I had faced had made me stronger. They had forced me to confront my vulnerabilities and to make changes that improved my quality of life. They had brought my family closer together and had given me a new perspective on the importance of self-care and resilience.

As I looked to the future, I was filled with a sense of hope and determination. I knew that there would be challenges, but I also knew that I had the strength and support to overcome them. The experience of battling pancreatitis, staph infection, E. coli, and pneumonia had made me stronger, and I was ready to continue thriving in life.

Chapter 7: The Power of Family

In my journey through life's challenges, the importance of family has been a constant source of strength and support. Among my family members, my sister Stacy and my niece Courtney have played pivotal roles in helping me navigate the trials and tribulations that came my way. Their unwavering love and encouragement have been instrumental in my journey to recovery and thriving.

Stacy has always been a guiding force in my life. As the eldest sibling, she took on the role of caregiver after our parents passed away, ensuring that our family remained intact and supported. Her resilience and determination were evident from a young age, and she quickly became the backbone of our family. Stacy's ability to balance work, family, and her own personal challenges was nothing short of remarkable.

When I was diagnosed with diabetes, Stacy was the first to step up and take charge. She meticulously researched diabetes management, learning about dietary changes, exercise routines, and medication options. Her dedication to my health was unwavering, and she made it her mission to ensure that I had the best possible care and support. From meal planning to attending doctor's appointments with me, Stacy was always by my side, offering guidance and encouragement.

Courtney, my niece, brought a different kind of support into my life. Her youthful energy and optimism were a breath of fresh air during some of the most challenging times. Courtney had a way of making even the toughest days a little brighter with her infectious laughter and boundless enthusiasm. She was always eager to help, whether it was preparing meals, organizing my medications, or simply spending time with me to lift my spirits.

During my stay at Emory University Hospital, Courtney's visits became a highlight of my days. She would bring books to read together, sharing stories that transported us to different worlds and provided a much-needed escape from the hospital environment. Courtney also introduced me to various foods, tempting my appetite and helping me maintain my nutrition during my recovery. Her efforts to keep my spirits high were deeply appreciated, and they played a crucial role in my healing process.

Stacy's support extended beyond my physical health. She understood the emotional toll that my medical conditions took on me and made it a point to be there for me in every way possible.

We would have long conversations about life, our dreams, and our fears. Stacy's wisdom and empathy were a source of comfort, and her belief in my ability to overcome my challenges gave me the strength to keep going.

The bond between Stacy and Courtney was also a testament to the power of family. Together, they formed a support network that was both strong and nurturing. Their teamwork and dedication to my well-being were inspiring, and they demonstrated the true meaning of family. Whether it was coordinating care, providing emotional support, or simply being there to listen, Stacy and Courtney worked together seamlessly to ensure that I had everything I needed.

One of the most memorable moments during my recovery was a surprise celebration organized by Stacy and Courtney. They invited family and friends to the hospital to celebrate a milestone in my healing journey. The room was filled with laughter, music, and heartfelt messages of encouragement. It was a reminder of the incredible support system I had and the importance of celebrating even the smallest victories.

Stacy's resilience was particularly evident during the times when I faced setbacks. Whether it was managing complications from my heart attack or battling infections during my stay at Emory, Stacy remained steadfast in her support. Her ability to stay calm and focused in the face of adversity was a source of strength for all of us. Stacy's determination to see me through these challenges was a testament to her unwavering love and commitment.

Courtney's youthful optimism and creativity also played a significant role in my recovery.

She often came up with fun activities and projects to keep me engaged and motivated. From art sessions to movie nights, Courtney found ways to bring joy and positivity into my life. Her presence was a constant reminder of the beauty and resilience of youth.

The support I received from Stacy and Courtney extended beyond the confines of the hospital. Once I was discharged and returned home, they continued to provide the care and encouragement I needed to thrive. Stacy helped me establish a routine that included healthy eating, regular exercise, and stress management. Courtney continued to bring her infectious energy and creativity into my daily life, making each day a little brighter.

Their unwavering support also had a profound impact on my mental and emotional well-being. The journey to recovery was not just about physical health; it was also about finding hope and purpose. Stacy and Courtney helped me rediscover my passions and encouraged me to pursue activities that brought me joy and fulfillment. Their belief in my ability to overcome my challenges was a powerful motivator and gave me the confidence to keep pushing forward.

The experience of navigating health challenges with the support of Stacy and Courtney also deepened my appreciation for the importance of family. I realized that family is not just about shared bloodlines but about the love, care, and support we provide for each other. Stacy and Courtney demonstrated the true meaning of family through their unwavering dedication and selflessness.

Reflecting on my journey, I am filled with gratitude for the incredible support I received from Stacy and Courtney. Their love, encouragement, and belief in my ability to overcome my challenges were instrumental in my recovery and continued well-being. The bond we share is a testament to the power of family and the resilience of the human spirit.

As I look to the future, I am inspired by the strength and love of Stacy and Courtney. Their support has given me the foundation to continue thriving and to face whatever challenges may come my way. The lessons I have learned from their unwavering dedication will stay with me forever, and I am committed to living my life with the same level of resilience and compassion that they have shown me.

The journey of healing and recovery is never easy, but with the support of family, it becomes a little more manageable. Stacy and Courtney have shown me the true meaning of family, and their love and support have been a guiding light in my life. Together, we have faced the challenges and celebrated the victories, and our bond has only grown stronger through it all.

Chapter 8: Brotherly Love

Throughout my journey, my older twin brothers, Bilal and Meco, have been my constant companions and sources of strength. Their unwavering support, loyalty, and love have played a significant role in my life, especially during the most challenging times. Bilal and Meco have stood by me as brothers in arms, facing every obstacle together and celebrating every victory.

Bilal, the elder twin by mere minutes, has always been a steady presence in my life. His calm demeanor and wisdom have guided me through many difficult situations. Bilal's ability to see the bigger picture and his pragmatic approach to life have been invaluable. He has a way of keeping things in perspective and providing sound advice when I needed it most.

Meco, on the other hand, brings a vibrant energy that complements Bilal's calmness. His enthusiasm, optimism, and adventurous spirit are infectious. Meco has a knack for finding joy in the simplest things and reminding us to appreciate the beauty of life. His positive outlook and unwavering support have been a source of inspiration for me.

Growing up, Bilal and Meco were inseparable. Their bond as twins was unique, and they shared an understanding that only twins could. This bond extended to me, and I always felt a deep sense of connection and camaraderie with them. Whether it was playing basketball in the park or tackling school projects, we were a team, and their presence provided a sense of security and belonging.

When I was diagnosed with diabetes, Bilal and Meco were there every step of the way. Bilal took on the role of researcher, delving into medical literature and providing valuable insights into diabetes management. He helped me understand the complexities of the condition and offered practical advice on how to navigate the challenges. Meco focused on keeping my spirits high. His humor and lightheartedness provided much-needed relief from the stress and anxiety of dealing with a chronic illness.

During my heart attack, the twins once again stepped up to support me. Bilal's calm and composed nature helped to steady my nerves during the emergency. He coordinated with the medical staff, ensuring that I received the best possible care. Meco, with his boundless energy, kept my spirits high during my recovery. He organized activities and outings that helped me stay active and engaged, even during the toughest days.

The bond between the three of us grew even stronger during my battle with pancreatitis. The pain and setbacks were overwhelming, but Bilal and Meco were always there to lift me up. Bilal's practical advice and Meco's infectious positivity were a powerful combination that kept me going. Their presence in the hospital, along with Stacy and Courtney, created a support network that was both strong and nurturing.

Bilal's resilience and determination have always been a source of inspiration for me. He faced his own challenges with grace and tenacity, and his ability to overcome obstacles has taught me valuable lessons. Bilal's support extended beyond practical help; he also provided emotional and mental strength that was crucial in my recovery. His belief in my ability to overcome my health challenges was unwavering, and it gave me the confidence to keep pushing forward.

Meco's youthful energy and adventurous spirit were a constant source of motivation. He found ways to make even the most mundane activities exciting and enjoyable. From organizing family game nights to planning weekend outings, Meco kept my spirits high and reminded me of the importance of finding joy in everyday life. His optimism and enthusiasm were a beacon of hope during some of the darkest moments.

One of the most memorable moments with Bilal and Meco was a weekend getaway they organized to celebrate my progress in recovery. They planned a trip to the mountains, where we spent time hiking, fishing, and simply enjoying the beauty of nature. The trip was a reminder of the strength of our bond and the importance of taking time to recharge and appreciate the simple pleasures in life.

The support I received from Bilal and Meco extended beyond my physical health. They understood the emotional toll that my medical conditions took on me and made it a point to be there for me in every way possible. We had countless conversations about life, our dreams, and our fears. Their empathy and understanding were a source of comfort, and their belief in my ability to overcome my challenges gave me the strength to keep going.

Reflecting on my journey, I am filled with gratitude for the incredible support I received from Bilal and Meco. Their love, encouragement, and belief in my ability to overcome my challenges were instrumental in my recovery and continued well-being. The bond we share is a testament to the power of family and the resilience of the human spirit.

As I look to the future, I am inspired by the strength and love of Bilal and Meco. Their support has given me the foundation to continue thriving and to face whatever challenges may come my way. The lessons I have learned from their unwavering dedication will stay with me forever, and I am committed to living my life with the same level of resilience and compassion that they have shown me.

The journey of healing and recovery is never easy, but with the support of family, it becomes a little more manageable. Bilal and Meco have shown me the true meaning of brotherhood, and their love and support have been a guiding light in my life. Together, we have faced the challenges and celebrated the victories, and our bond has only grown stronger through it all.

Chapter 9: Strength and Resilience

My journey through life's challenges has been a testament to the incredible strength and resilience of my family. Among my family members, Charity, Kathy, and many others have played pivotal roles in providing the support, love, and encouragement that have helped me navigate life's ups and downs. Their unwavering dedication and belief in my ability to overcome challenges have been instrumental in my journey to recovery and thriving.

Charity's presence in my life has been a beacon of hope and positivity. Her compassionate nature and genuine concern for my well-being have made her an essential part of my support system. Charity has always been there for me, whether it was during my health struggles or everyday life challenges. Her dedication to ensuring that I had everything I needed was a testament to her selflessness and love.

One of the most memorable moments with Charity was during my stay at Emory University Hospital. Charity would visit me regularly, bringing books and different foods to keep me engaged and nourished. Her visits were a highlight of my days, providing a much-needed distraction from the pain and monotony of hospital life. We would spend hours reading together, sharing stories and discussing various topics. Charity's efforts to keep my spirits high were deeply appreciated and played a crucial role in my healing process.

Charity's support extended beyond the hospital. When I returned home, she continued to be a constant presence, helping me with my recovery and ensuring that I stayed on track with my health goals. Charity's dedication to my well-being was unwavering, and her belief in my ability to overcome my challenges was a powerful motivator. Her love and encouragement gave me the strength to keep pushing forward, even on the toughest days.

Chapter 10: A New Beginning for Antonio

Antonio Champion, a 48-year-old man, has recently faced some of the most significant health challenges of his life. Suffering from a heart attack, diabetes, and pancreatitis, Antonio's journey towards recovery and a healthier lifestyle has just begun. This chapter explores the changes and management strategies he must embrace to improve his overall health and well-being.

The Turning Point

Antonio's heart attack was a wake-up call, reminding him of the fragility of life and the importance of taking care of his body. The event not only highlighted the need for immediate medical intervention but also underscored the necessity of long-term lifestyle changes. Antonio knew that to prevent future complications, he had to make significant adjustments to his daily habits.

Heart Health Management

1. Quitting Smoking: Antonio had been a smoker for over two decades. Quitting smoking was the first and most crucial step in his recovery. With the help of nicotine replacement therapy and support groups, Antonio began his journey towards a smoke-free life.

2. Adopting a Heart-Healthy Diet: Antonio's diet needed a complete overhaul. He replaced processed foods with whole grains, lean proteins, and an abundance of fruits and vegetables. By avoiding trans fats, high-sodium foods, and sugary snacks, he aimed to lower his cholesterol and blood pressure.

3. Regular Exercise: Incorporating regular physical activity into his routine was essential. Antonio started with daily walks and gradually included swimming and light weight training. These activities helped strengthen his heart and improve his cardiovascular health.

4. Medication Adherence: Following his heart attack, Antonio was prescribed medications to manage his condition. Consistently taking these medications and attending regular follow-up appointments with his cardiologist were vital components of his recovery plan.

Diabetes Management

1. Understanding Blood Sugar Levels: Antonio learned the importance of monitoring his blood sugar levels. Using a glucometer, he regularly checked his levels to ensure they remained within the target range.

2. Nutrition and Diet Adjustments: Managing diabetes required careful attention to his diet. Antonio focused on carbohydrate counting and meal planning. He incorporated a variety of nutrient-dense foods while avoiding sugary drinks and high-calorie snacks.

3. Physical Activity and Diabetes: Regular exercise played a dual role in Antonio's life. Not only did it improve his heart health, but it also helped regulate his blood sugar levels. He aimed for at least 150 minutes of aerobic activity each week.

4. Medication and Insulin Management: Antonio was prescribed medications and insulin to manage his diabetes. Understanding how to administer insulin and adjusting doses based on his blood sugar readings were crucial for maintaining control over his condition.

Pancreatitis Management

1. Dietary Changes for Pancreatitis: Antonio's pancreatitis required a low-fat diet. He avoided greasy foods, high-fat dairy products, and alcohol. Instead, he opted for lean proteins like chicken and fish, along with plenty of vegetables.

2. Pain Management Strategies: Dealing with the pain associated with pancreatitis was challenging. Antonio used a combination of over-the-counter pain relievers and alternative therapies like acupuncture and relaxation techniques.

3. Importance of Hydration: Staying hydrated was essential for managing pancreatitis. Antonio made it a habit to drink at least eight glasses of water a day and included hydrating foods like cucumbers and melons in his diet.

4. Regular Medical Check-Ups: Monitoring his pancreatic health through regular imaging tests and blood work was crucial. These check-ups allowed his healthcare providers to adjust his treatment plan as needed.

Integrative Approach to Health Management

1. Coordinating Care with Healthcare Providers: Antonio understood the importance of building a support team. His healthcare providers included a primary care physician, cardiologist, endocrinologist, and nutritionist. Effective communication among them was key to his integrated care.

2. Stress Management Techniques: Managing stress was an important aspect of Antonio's overall health. He practiced mindfulness meditation, deep breathing exercises, and gentle yoga to reduce stress levels.

3. Importance of Sleep and Rest: Antonio prioritized sleep hygiene by maintaining a regular sleep schedule and creating a restful environment. Adequate rest improved his mental clarity and mood.

Antonio's journey towards a healthier lifestyle was not easy, but his determination and commitment were unwavering. By making these comprehensive lifestyle changes and working closely with his healthcare team, Antonio took control of his health and paved the way for a brighter, healthier future.

His story is a testament to the power of resilience and the human spirit. It serves as an inspiration to others facing similar challenges, reminding them that with the right mindset and support, it is possible to overcome even the most daunting health obstacles.

Antonio's Daily Routine for Health Management

To better understand how Antonio incorporates these lifestyle changes and management strategies into his daily life, let's take a closer look at his typical day.

Morning Routine

Antonio starts his day early, around 6:00 AM, to ensure he has enough time to manage his health before heading to work.

1. Mindfulness and Meditation: Antonio begins with a 10-minute mindfulness meditation session to set a positive tone for the day. This practice helps him manage stress and focus on the present moment.

2. Healthy Breakfast: He enjoys a heart-healthy breakfast that includes oatmeal topped with fresh berries, a slice of whole-grain toast,

and a cup of green tea. This meal is low in fat and high in fiber, providing the energy he needs to kickstart his day.

3. Medication and Blood Sugar Monitoring: After breakfast, Antonio takes his prescribed medications for his heart and diabetes. He also checks his blood sugar levels to ensure they are within the target range.

4. Light Exercise: Antonio incorporates light exercise into his morning routine. He usually goes for a 30-minute brisk walk around his neighborhood. This activity helps improve his cardiovascular health and manage his blood sugar levels.

Workday Habits

As Antonio heads to work, he continues to prioritize his health throughout the day.

1. Healthy Snacking: Antonio keeps healthy snacks like nuts, yogurt, and fruit at his desk to avoid unhealthy temptations. These snacks help maintain his blood sugar levels and provide sustained energy.

2. Hydration: He carries a reusable water bottle and drinks water regularly to stay hydrated, especially important for managing his pancreatitis.

3. Stress Management: During his lunch break, Antonio takes a few minutes to practice deep breathing exercises or take a short walk to reduce stress and clear his mind.

4. Balanced Lunch: Antonio enjoys a balanced lunch that includes a lean protein source, such as grilled chicken or fish, along with a variety of vegetables and a whole-grain side. He avoids high-fat and high-sugar foods that could negatively impact his health.

Evening Routine

Antonio's evening routine is designed to help him relax and prepare for a restful night's sleep.

1. Dinner Preparation: After work, Antonio prepares a healthy dinner with his family. They often cook together, choosing recipes that are low in fat and high in nutrients. A typical dinner might include a baked salmon fillet, quinoa, and steamed broccoli.

2. Post-Dinner Walk: Antonio and his family take a leisurely walk after dinner. This not only helps with digestion but also provides an opportunity for family bonding.

3. Medication and Blood Sugar Monitoring: Before bed, Antonio takes his evening medications and checks his blood sugar levels again. This routine helps him maintain

control over his diabetes and ensures his body is in good shape overnight.

4. Relaxation and Sleep: To wind down, Antonio reads a book or listens to calming music. He aims for at least 7-8 hours of sleep each night, which is essential for his overall health and well-being.

Support System and Community

Antonio's journey towards better health is supported by a strong network of family, friends, and healthcare providers.

1. Family Involvement: Antonio's family plays a crucial role in his health management. They support his dietary changes, join him in physical activities, and encourage him to stay on track with his medications and medical appointments.

2. Healthcare Team: Regular check-ups with his healthcare providers ensure that Antonio's treatment plans are effective and adjusted as needed. Open communication with his primary care physician, cardiologist, endocrinologist, and nutritionist is vital for coordinated care.

3. Support Groups: Antonio participates in local support groups for individuals with similar health conditions. These groups provide a sense of community, share valuable tips, and offer emotional support.

Reflections on Progress

Antonio's commitment to his health has yielded significant improvements. He feels more energetic, has better control over his blood sugar levels, and experiences fewer episodes of pain from pancreatitis. Most importantly, he has reduced his risk of future heart attacks and is living a more fulfilling life.

Antonio's story is a powerful reminder that with determination, support, and the right strategies, it is possible to overcome health challenges and make lasting positive changes. His journey serves as an inspiration to others facing similar obstacles, proving that a healthier, happier life is within reach.

In conclusion, Antonio's transformation is a testament to the power of lifestyle changes and effective health management. By quitting smoking, adopting a heart-healthy diet, engaging in regular exercise, and managing his medications, Antonio has taken control of his health. His commitment to monitoring his blood sugar levels, following a low-fat diet, and staying hydrated has helped him manage his diabetes and pancreatitis. With the support of his family, healthcare team, and community, Antonio continues to strive for a healthier future.

Conclusion: Reflection and Future Outlook

Reflection on Antonio's Journey

Antonio's journey towards better health has been marked by determination, resilience, and an unwavering commitment to change. Facing multiple health challenges, including a heart attack, diabetes, and pancreatitis, Antonio had to make significant lifestyle adjustments and embrace a holistic approach to health management. This reflection will delve into the key aspects of his journey and the lessons learned along the way.

1. The Importance of Early Intervention and Lifestyle Changes

Antonio's heart attack served as a pivotal moment, highlighting the urgent need for lifestyle modifications. He realized that early intervention and proactive health management could significantly reduce the risk of future complications. By quitting smoking, adopting a heart-healthy diet, and incorporating regular exercise into his routine, Antonio took crucial steps towards improving his cardiovascular health.

2. The Role of Comprehensive Diabetes Management

Managing diabetes required Antonio to pay close attention to his diet, exercise, and medication regimen. He learned the importance of monitoring blood sugar levels, counting carbohydrates, and staying physically active.

Antonio's dedication to these practices helped him achieve better control over his diabetes and reduce the risk of related complications.

3. Coping with Pancreatitis

Pancreatitis posed its own set of challenges, requiring Antonio to follow a strict low-fat diet and avoid alcohol. Managing pain and staying hydrated were also critical components of his care. Through regular check-ups and open communication with his healthcare providers, Antonio successfully navigated the complexities of this condition.

4. The Power of a Support System

Antonio's journey was not one he faced alone. His family, healthcare providers, and support groups played an integral role in his success. Their encouragement, guidance, and emotional support were invaluable in helping Antonio stay motivated and focused on his health goals.

5. Embracing a Holistic Approach

Antonio's experience underscored the importance of a holistic approach to health management. Beyond physical health, he also prioritized mental and emotional well-being through mindfulness, meditation, and stress management techniques. This integrative approach contributed to his overall sense of balance and fulfillment.

Future Outlook and Goals

As Antonio looks to the future, his focus remains on maintaining and building upon the progress he has made. The following goals outline his path forward:

1. Sustaining Healthy Habits

Antonio is committed to sustaining the healthy habits he has developed. This includes continuing to follow a balanced diet, engaging in regular physical activity, and adhering to his medication regimen. By maintaining these practices, Antonio aims to further reduce his risk of heart disease, manage his diabetes effectively, and prevent pancreatitis flare-ups.

2. Enhancing Physical Fitness

While Antonio has made significant strides in incorporating exercise into his routine, he plans to enhance his physical fitness by exploring new activities. Whether it's taking up a new sport, joining a fitness class, or embarking on outdoor adventures, Antonio is excited to challenge himself and improve his overall fitness levels.

3. Strengthening Mental and Emotional Well-Being

Antonio recognizes the importance of mental and emotional health in his overall well-being. He intends to continue practicing mindfulness and meditation, while also exploring other relaxation techniques like yoga and tai chi. Antonio is also open to seeking professional counseling or therapy if needed, to address any emotional challenges that may arise.

4. Building a Stronger Support Network

Antonio plans to strengthen his support network by staying connected with his healthcare providers and participating in support groups. He also aims to foster deeper connections with friends and family, creating a community of support that can help him navigate any future health challenges.

5. Setting and Achieving New Health Goals

Antonio's journey has taught him the value of setting achievable health goals. Moving forward, he will continue to set specific, measurable, and realistic goals for his health and well-being. Whether it's reaching a new fitness milestone, achieving a healthier weight, or managing his conditions more effectively, Antonio is determined to keep striving for improvement.

6. Inspiring Others

Antonio's story is a powerful testament to the impact of lifestyle changes and proactive health management. He hopes to inspire others facing similar health challenges to take charge of their own well-being. By sharing his experiences and the lessons he has learned, Antonio aims to motivate and support others on their own journeys towards better health.

Antonio's Commitment to Long-Term Health

Antonio's commitment to his long-term health involves not just maintaining the changes he has made but continuously striving for improvement. His journey is a dynamic process, requiring ongoing attention and adaptability.

Continued Education and Awareness

Antonio understands the importance of staying informed about his health conditions. He regularly reads up-to-date literature on heart health, diabetes management, and pancreatitis care. By keeping himself educated, Antonio can make informed decisions and adapt his lifestyle as new information becomes available.

Setting Realistic and Achievable Goals

Antonio's journey is marked by setting realistic and achievable goals. He uses the SMART criteria (Specific, Measurable, Achievable, Relevant, Time-bound) to define his health objectives. For instance, he might set a goal to walk 10,000 steps daily, reduce his HbA1c levels by a certain percentage, or prepare a new healthy recipe each week.

Celebrating Milestones

Celebrating milestones is an integral part of Antonio's journey. Whether it's reaching a weight loss target, achieving a new fitness goal, or successfully managing his blood sugar levels, Antonio takes the time to acknowledge and celebrate his achievements. These celebrations provide motivation and reinforce positive behavior.

Adapting to Challenges

Life is full of challenges, and Antonio's journey is no exception. He has learned to adapt to setbacks and view them as opportunities for growth. Whether it's dealing with a temporary rise in blood sugar levels or managing a flare-up of pancreatitis, Antonio approaches each challenge with a problem-solving mindset. He consults his healthcare providers, adjusts his treatment plans, and remains resilient.

Leveraging Technology

Antonio leverages technology to support his health management. He uses smartphone apps to track his diet, exercise, and blood sugar levels. These tools provide valuable insights and help him stay on track. Additionally, Antonio participates in online support groups and forums where he connects with others facing similar health challenges.

Inspirational Message for Others

Antonio's story is a beacon of hope and inspiration for others facing similar health challenges. His journey demonstrates that with dedication, support, and the right strategies, it is possible to overcome health obstacles and lead a fulfilling life. Antonio's experience serves as a reminder that positive change is within reach for everyone.

1. Believe in Yourself

Antonio's journey began with a belief in his ability to change. Self-belief is a powerful motivator, and it can inspire others to take the first step towards better health. Antonio encourages others to believe in their own potential and capabilities.

2. Seek Support

No one has to face health challenges alone. Antonio's support system was instrumental in his success. He advises others to seek support from family, friends, healthcare providers, and support groups. Building a network of support can provide encouragement, guidance, and accountability.

3. Embrace Change

Change can be daunting, but it is also empowering. Antonio embraced the changes necessary to improve his health, and he encourages others to do the same. Whether it's adopting a healthier diet, quitting smoking, or incorporating exercise into daily life, small changes can make a significant difference.

4. Stay Informed

Knowledge is a powerful tool in health management. Antonio's commitment to staying informed helped him make better decisions and adapt to new information. He encourages others to educate themselves about their health conditions and stay updated on the latest advancements.

5. Celebrate Progress

Celebrating progress, no matter how small, is essential. Antonio's milestones provided motivation and reinforced his commitment to his health goals. He advises others to acknowledge and celebrate their achievements, as each step forward is a testament to their dedication and hard work.

6. Adapt and Persevere

Health journeys are rarely linear. Antonio's ability to adapt to challenges and persevere through setbacks was crucial to his success. He encourages others to view obstacles as opportunities for growth and to remain resilient in the face of adversity.

A Brighter Future

As Antonio looks to the future, his vision is filled with hope and optimism. He is committed to maintaining his healthy lifestyle and continuing his journey towards better health. Antonio's story is a testament to the transformative power of determination, support, and a holistic approach to health management.

Continuing the Journey

Antonio's journey is ongoing, and he remains dedicated to his health and well-being. He looks forward to exploring new activities, setting new goals, and inspiring others along the way. Antonio's story is a reminder that positive change is possible and that a brighter, healthier future is within reach for everyone.

Conclusion

Antonio Champion's journey from a heart attack, diabetes, and pancreatitis to a healthier, more fulfilling life is a powerful testament to the impact of lifestyle changes and proactive health management. His story underscores the importance of early intervention, comprehensive care, and a holistic approach to well-being. As Antonio continues to navigate his health journey, his commitment to maintaining healthy habits, enhancing his fitness, and prioritizing mental and emotional health will guide him towards a brighter future. Antonio's experience serves as an inspiration to others, proving that with dedication, support, and the right strategies, positive change is possible.

Made in the USA
Columbia, SC
13 April 2025